Practical tips for Baby hacks

simple tips to make life easier

Shahnaz Afroj Tuli.

The author's bio

I, Shahnaz Afroj Tuli, am a Bangladeshi writer. I got a Master's degree in Botany from National University. As far back as I can remember, I've always wanted to put pen to paper. My main interest is writing.

 The role of parents in society is crucial. From what I've seen, strong parenting skills are something everyone should have some understanding of. It is my sincere hope that this book will be of service to you.

Table of Contents

Introduction

I've always wanted to be a mom since I became a woman. When I see a baby, my heart starts to melt. It's essential to know how to raise your children, from before you get pregnant to after you give birth. This is important for the new mother and the whole family.

Family is vital to us. Without it, we wouldn't be worth much. However, we need to prepare for motherhood for it to go well.

Getting ready ahead of time

If you know ahead of time what happens to the body and mind during each trimester, many things won't seem strange.
Education about the physical and emotional changes, watching videos about it, talking to someone who has given birth, mentally preparing yourself that it's only a matter of days, thinking about who will be available if needed and who will help with what." These things help you get ready for pregnancy.

Pregnant women should eat a healthy, well-balanced diet.When a woman is pregnant, it can be excruciating if the people around her don't try to understand her.The most important thing is to get help, especially from the husband.

"A child of a mother is not just one child. Two youngsters. If the mother doesn't care for herself and her mental health problems, her unborn child will be hurt. Husbands need to realize that their wives' health affects their children's health. They shouldn't do anything that could hurt a woman who is pregnant. stress."

Chapter:01

When a woman is pregnant, almost every part of her body changes...

When a woman is pregnant and carries the baby in her womb for nine months or more, the heart, brain, arms, legs, and other organs slowly change into a fetus.At the same time, both the bodies and minds of women started to change in different ways.

The changes that happen in a woman's body during pregnancy are caused by two hormones called estrogen and progesterone. The first three months don't show any changes on the outside.

Many pregnant women feel sick in the early stages, especially in the morning. Because of this, you can't eat. And what everyone does is gain weight. For normal pregnant women is to gain up to 2 kg per month, or up to 15 kg over the course of their pregnancy.

During pregnancy, a woman's bones loosen up at the joints.

The backbone is pushed down by a heavy stomach or a bigger front of the body. There could be back pain. Gestational diabetes is a term for when a woman is pregnant and has high blood sugar. Usually, it goes away after the baby is born.

The gums may swell up, bleed when you brush your teeth, or hurt.As the uterus gets bigger, it puts pressure on the urinary bladder. So they have to go to the bathroom a lot. As the size of the uterus grows, the lungs can't expand enough. So many people might have trouble breathing.

During pregnancy, there is a chance of anemia because the body needs more iron. During this time, a woman's body makes more fluid than usual. This can cause water to build up in the legs and make them swell.

High blood pressure is common.Hormones make the breasts bigger and darken the area around the nipple. The baby can feed from the breast now. Many people have pain in their breasts.Lactogen is a hormone that helps make breast milk.There may be more interest in sex.Or it could stop growing altogether.

White discharge may come out of the vagina, and bleeding may happen, but you don't need to worry if it's not too much.When a woman is pregnant, her feelings change in significant ways.These are the main changes to your body when you're pregnant, which are different for each woman.

The hormone oxytocin makes the uterus contract after birth.But a lot of things don't go back to where they were. For example, many people still have trouble with their weight, stretch marks, and diabetes.

How something affects the mind

All these changes in their bodies cause a lot of stress in their minds.Women's minds are full of worry, uncertainty, sadness, anger, and mood swings.Many people can't keep their feelings in check. They don't cry much, get upset, angry, or irritable.

A pregnant woman's moods change a lot because she has no control over them. One day she feels good, and the next day she feels bad. Her body's changing state affects her mental health, and she can't do much when she wants to. This makes her feel trapped.Pregnant women need a lot of help from their friends and family.

The fear of the unknown, not knowing how the nine months of pregnancy will go, not knowing if the baby will be healthy, not knowing if family. Friends will help, and adjusting to this significant change in life often causes stress, anxiety, and depression.

Chapter:02

Food that women who are pregnant should eat

Every child in the world needs a mother, like a banyan tree. Children grow up safe and secure with their mother's endless affection and love. So, the first thing to look at is the mother's diet.

Taking good care of the mother-to-be is the most important thing for a healthy, standard delivery. Terrible things can happen in the first three months of pregnancy. Many pregnant women feel sick during this time, don't want to eat, lose weight, and get anaemia. So the family members should ensure good health and a balanced diet for the expectant mother. Especially from five months onwards, the mother's diet should be balanced for the proper growth of the fetus, with meat, calcium, vitamins, minerals and enough water. Also, ensure adequate sleep or rest.

For instance, the Food and Nutrition Board of the United States says pregnant women should eat 20 grams more meat than they need during the last two months of their pregnancy. These foods that aren't vegetables are best if they come from animals. The food also has an extra 500 mg calcium and 5 mg iron. They suggest consuming enough milk and nuts to meet the calcium requirement.

Aside from this, osteomalacia is a bone disease caused by insufficient calcium and vitamin D. Aside from this, the pregnant woman should eat things like sea fish that have iodine in them because a child needs iodine for their brain and intelligence to grow. In the early stages of pregnancy, the baby's weight grows by 1 gram daily. After five months, however, it starts to grow by 10 grams per day. In the last two months of pregnancy, half of the baby's total weight increases. For this reason, the mother's diet should be given extra attention.

Diet:

From 8:30 a.m. to 8:30 a.m., four or two pieces of bread, one egg, and two cups of vegetables. 11 a.m. to 11:30 a.m.: 250 mg of milk or 60 g of nuts, two biscuits or crackers, and any seasonal fruit. Lunch: three cups of rice (in a medium cup of tea), two pieces of fish or meat, one day a week of seafood, vegetables, salad, lemon, and one cup of pulses. 5 p.m. to 6 p.m.: 250 mg of milk or soup or 60 g of nuts, biscuits, crackers, or one cup of noodles. Night: four cups of rice, at least two pieces of fish or meat, seafood once a week, vegetables, and one cup of pulses.

Some common misunderstandings about food: Many of the older people in the house tell the mother-to-be not to overeat. They think that giving the baby more food will help it grow. And you have to have a cesarean when you get older. Because of this, the mother becomes malnourished, and the baby is born too small and too young.

This is not at all true. Besides, the mother is given the wrong idea about some nutritious foods. For instance, if a child eats an epileptic fish, it can cause seizures. When kids eat boal fish, their jaws get bigger.

When a child eats horn or shoal fish, their body changes into a snake. People say that if a child eats cucumbers, the skin on their body will crack. Eating a banana will make you cold. Mother is not allowed to eat during a lunar eclipse or a solar eclipse. Etc. There are many false ideas, which are just that. It is also a reason why mothers don't get enough to eat.

Some tips:

- Eat well-balanced food and stay away from certain raw foods.

- Pregnant women can walk and work out regularly.

- Pregnant women should sleep on their backs instead of their sides.

- If there are no problems, you should see your doctor at least four times during pregnancy.

- They are taking folic acid and calcium as the doctor told them to
- Brush your teeth every day.

- Add things you like, hobbies, and things that make you feel at peace with your life.

Chapter:03

Food that women who are pregnant should eat

Every child in the world needs a mother, like a banyan tree. Children grow up safe and secure with their mother's endless affection and love. So, the first thing to look at is the mother's diet.

Taking good care of the mother-to-be is the most important thing for a healthy, standard delivery. Terrible things can happen in the first three months of pregnancy. Many pregnant women feel sick during this time, don't want to eat, lose weight, and get anaemia. So the family members should ensure good health and a balanced diet for the expectant mother. Especially from five months onwards, the mother's diet should be balanced for the proper growth of the fetus, with meat, calcium, vitamins, minerals and enough water. Also, ensure adequate sleep or rest.

For instance, the Food and Nutrition Board of the United States says pregnant women should eat 20 grams more meat than they need during the last two months of their pregnancy. These foods that aren't vegetables are best if they come from animals. The food also has an extra 500 mg calcium and 5 mg iron. They suggest consuming enough milk and nuts to meet the calcium requirement.

Aside from this, osteomalacia is a bone disease caused by insufficient calcium and vitamin D. Aside from this, the pregnant woman should eat things like sea fish that have iodine in them because a child needs iodine for their brain and intelligence to grow. In the early stages of pregnancy, the baby's weight grows by 1 gram daily. After five months, however, it starts to grow by 10 grams per day. In the last two months of pregnancy, half of the baby's total weight increases. For this reason, the mother's diet should be given extra attention.

Diet: From 8:30 a.m. to 8:30 a.m., four or two pieces of bread, one egg, and two cups of vegetables. 11 a.m. to 11:30 a.m.: 250 mg of milk or 60 g of nuts, two biscuits or crackers, and any seasonal fruit. Lunch: three cups of rice (in a medium cup of tea), two pieces of fish or meat, one day a week of seafood, vegetables, salad, lemon, and one cup of pulses. 5 p.m. to 6 p.m.: 250 mg of milk or soup or 60 g of nuts, biscuits, crackers, or one cup of noodles. Night: four cups of rice, at least two pieces of fish or meat, seafood once a week, vegetables, and one cup of pulses.

Some common misunderstandings about food: Many of the older people in the house tell the mother-to-be not to overeat. They think that giving the baby more food will help it grow. And you have to have a cesarean when you get older. Because of this, the mother becomes malnourished, and the baby is born too small and too young. This is not at all true. Besides, the mother is given the wrong idea about some nutritious foods. For instance, if a child eats an epileptic fish, it can cause seizures.

When kids eat boal fish, their jaws get bigger. When a child eats horn or shoal fish, their body changes into a snake. People say that if a child eats cucumbers, the skin on their body will crack. Eating a banana will make you cold. Mother is prohibited from eating during a lunar eclipse or a solar eclipse. Etc. There are many false ideas, which are just that. It is also a reason why mothers don't get enough to eat.

Chapter:04

When the baby comes into the world

After 36 or 37 weeks of pregnancy, it's a good idea to start getting ready in your mind for the birth. During these preparations, one of the most important things to consider is how the mother-to-be will know when it's time to give birth. At this time, the uterus may contract, which may cause a little pain in the lower abdomen. However, the mother will only feel the signs of labour or delivery if she knows them. Or you might not have time to go to the hospital. This can lead to several problems. What are the signs that labour is going well?

* Having lower-abdominal pain and contractions of the uterus

* Blood-tinged discharge

*The cervix opens up

* Getting a watery sac

Pains that feel like labour can happen late in pregnancy, especially 1-2 weeks before the due date. It isn't real work. When the uterus contracts after 16 weeks of pregnancy, these are called Braxton Hicks contractions. But there is no pain with it. There are some signs that a woman is in labour. Pain will start regularly, and the uterus will contract, which means the abdomen will get tighter. Over time, the pain's intensity and length will get worse. The pain won't always be there. But the time between them will get shorter and shorter over time. The pain starts in the back and moves through the thigh to the front. Neither painkillers nor sleeping pills help at all.

In false labour pain or false labour, the pain is less severe and only in the lower abdomen and groin. There are no contractions of the uterus or tightening of the stomach, and the pain can be treated with medicine.

The mucus covers the mouth of the uterus to protect the baby from getting sick from the outside. However, when the baby is born, this mouth opens, the water breaks, and a bloody fluid emerges. This is a vital sign that labour is about to start. But if any of those things happen, the pregnant woman should be taken to the hospital immediately because the baby could come anytime after the labour begins.

Postnatal care

Postnatal care includes regular health checks, good advice, and taking care of both the mother and the baby. A mother's health may be at risk after she has given birth. Because the mother's uterus and other reproductive organs take about 6 weeks to get back to normal after giving birth. This time is known as the "Pureperium."

During the puerperium, the mother needs to get care for her health.We need to focus some symtoms.

- Stopping perinatal infections is important.
- Making sure the mother stays healthy.
- To see if the baby is being fed by the mother or not.
- How to plan a family.
- Helping the mother and her family care for the child.
- Telling children how to get immunized.
- Postnatal care schedule.

Danger signs of the time after giving birth

- fever
- blood pressure too high
- Chest pain and trouble getting enough air
- Getting urine in the vaginal area
- Abdominal pain
- Foul-smelling discharge.
- Something falls into the genital area.

Chapter:05

Food for mothers

A child smiles as its mother holds it. Of course, the child will laugh if the mother does. The way a mother talks becomes a bully for her child. The child stops crying when the mother smiles and says a few loving words. This is a matter of what the eyes and ears see and hear. But it makes sense that what the mother eats affects what the baby eats when it is first born. Still, why aren't the health and nutrition of mothers being taken care of?

It takes a mother six weeks to feel like herself again after giving birth. The mother's energy, blood loss, and water needs should be met as best as possible. And the baby's body gets all kinds of nutrients from the mother's milk, like sugar, meat, and sweet foods. For the first six months, the baby doesn't need any other food or water. If the baby is given any other food during this time, it can cause several problems. Until the child is six months old, it gets all of its food from the mother. So the mother has no choice but to eat a healthy diet.

A mother needs a lot of water or liquid food when a baby is born. The mother should drink 4 to 4 and a half litres of fluid every day until her milk flow returns to normal (which may take approximately 15 to 2 months). After that, you only need to drink 2.5 to 3 litres of fluid daily. Before each meal, the mother will drink the liquid.

beginning few days

For the first three days after giving birth, the mother should drink lots of water. After that, there's chicken soup, jauvat, and red tea. For the first six weeks, you must eat a lot. Get plenty of meat. Eat milk, pulses, and vegetables with a lot of water (like a gourd, jali, and papaya) and foods high in calcium. The broth should be used to cook food. Soft rice can be eaten.

Calculating Calories

They were getting 400–500 more calories than usual every day until the last day of the pregnancy. Several things affect how this measurement is made. First, even people who eat meat want enough. In this way, six months had passed since the child's birth. After six months, the rule is to add more food to the baby's diet slowly. So, the mother's daily food intake can be cut to 200 calories in six months.

But this is just an average number. The number of calories a mother needs depends on how much milk the baby drinks and how fast the baby gains weight. The only way to figure out how many calories are needed is to know what is going on with the mother's body. So, you can't make rules set in stone until you know everything. For example, if the mother has diabetes, the food for the whole day should be broken up into several smaller meals.

Materials required

The needs for minerals and vitamins are the same as usual. Eat milk, fish, meat, and eggs. Essential fatty acids are also important. Fish should be eaten to ensure the baby's brain gets all the nutrients it needs (it is not right to throw away fish oil). You should eat fresh fruits and vegetables. If you eat foods high in fibre, you won't have trouble going to the bathroom.

Chapter:06

It is essential to keep young children from becoming malnourished.

To get enough nutrients and build a robust immune system, babies must be breastfed until they are six months old. Once the baby is six months old, he can start eating foods like cereal, vegetables, and eggs that the rest of the family eats. After that, a child should get breast milk and other foods from the family until they are two years old.

We call this "complementary feeding." This helps the baby get used to eating family food instead of breast milk. It is essential to give the baby the nutrition it needs as it grows. From six months to 24 months, a baby's nutritional needs are met, and he develops physically and mentally during this time.

The mother's breast milk must be given to the baby within an hour of birth. This milk has many components that keep babies from getting common illnesses like diarrhoea and pneumonia.

How to feed a baby

There are many different kinds of nutrients in a mother's milk. Aside from this, babies' yellow milk after birth is vital for keeping them from getting sick.Until six months old, babies can only and best eat breast milk. After six months, the baby needs foods other than breast milk to get all the nutrients and grow and develop normally. But until a baby is two years old, they don't need milk other than breast milk or colostrum. This is because there are many different nutrients in a mother's milk. Aside from this, babies' yellow milk after birth is essential for keeping them from getting sick.

Because breast milk is easy to digest, clean, and has anti-inflammatory properties, it makes it much less likely that your baby will get sick. As a result, breastfed babies are less likely to get asthma, lung diseases, obesity, type-1 diabetes, ear infections, stomach problems (like diarrhoea and vomiting), SIDS, etc.

In addition, mothers who breastfeed their babies are less likely to get high blood pressure, diabetes, breast cancer, and uterus cancer. But store-bought baby foods can't protect babies as well as their mothers' milk. Because of this, the chance of getting different diseases goes up.

When breastfeeding a newborn, it's important to remember the following:

For the baby's health, the mother must eat a well-balanced diet.The mother should drink one to two glasses of water or liquid food before each feeding.Feeding shouldn't be done quickly. It would be best if you ate slowly and with a calm mind.

If you want to sit down and feed your baby, put a pillow behind the mother's back and on her lap. If you want to feed your baby while lying down, the baby should be facing you so that you can hold the back of the baby with your hands.

Be careful not to put too much pressure on the baby's nose.

Feed well from one breast each time because thin milk comes out first and then thick milk.The baby should get breast milk every two hours. So even if you take a break for four hours straight while sleeping at night, there is no problem.

Working moms can store breast milk so their babies don't run out of milk while at work. If that's the case, pump and put the milk in the fridge every time you come home from work to feed the baby. But you can't give the child milk straight from the fridge because it's cold. So instead, put the milk bottle in a bowl of hot water and shake it to make it easier for the baby to drink.

If the mother has corona, wash her hands with soap and water, put on a mask, and feed the baby milk.

Chapter:07

Care for a baby

A newborn is a baby who is less than 28 days old. This time is essential for both the mother and the child. Cleanliness is the only thing that can keep babies safe. Her thin, soft body is elementary to handle.

They can get sick from different pathogens. The baby's first hour after birth is the most important. So, for the child, it is "Golden One Hour." After birth, the first and only thing to do is feed the baby the mother's milk (shalduh). Colostrum is like a baby's first shot of medicine. And it keeps the child from getting sick. Even though there isn't much milk, it gives the baby all the nutrition it needs. If a baby is fed milk, it is less likely to get night fever, jaundice, and other diseases. If both mom and baby drink milk, they will be healthy. Exclusive breastfeeding means the baby only gets breast milk for the first six months.

A soft cloth should be used to clean the baby after birth. It's the summer. No thick material should be used to cover the baby during this time. It might make the child antsy. However, it will do to wrap the baby in a light, soft cloth. A fan or AC can be turned on in the room if needed.

A baby should not be bathed for the first three days after birth. A new baby should weigh about 2.5 kg. If the baby weighs less than this or has any other problem, the doctor should be called.

Honey or sugar water should not be given to a baby right after birth. Instead, the mother should drink more water after the baby is born. Other than that, the mother should be able to eat the same food as the rest of the family.

Many people keep the doors and windows of the room where the baby stays from birth until they are 28 days old. This is never a good thing to do. Instead, the baby and the mother should be kept in a room with open doors and windows. So that light and air from outside can get into the house.

No one outside the family should pick up the baby. Because if someone comes in from the outside, he might be full of dirt and germs. When they hold the baby in their hands, they can spread germs to the baby. Because of this, the baby shouldn't be saved. If you have to take it, you can wash your hands with something that kills germs or use an instant hand sanitiser. Also, it would help if you washed your hands after changing a child's diaper or clothes wet with urine.

The nails of children increase. He might get hurt by his claws. Ulceration could happen if the scratch is deep. So cleanly cut the little nails. If you wait until the baby is asleep, you won't have to worry about moving or missing. And if you want to cut while awake, you should ask for help.

 But don't squeeze too hard Most children have soft nails.But if it feels hard, cut the nails after a shower.Pay attention to how comfortable and absorbent the clothes and diapers are when you dress the baby and choose them.

How to dress and keep clean

Give the child clean winter clothes and something to cover their head. Bathe the baby after at least three days. Every other day until the baby is one month old (winter time). After a month, you should wash it every day. Give the child a warm bath with the water you boil. It's OK to massage oil into your skin before you shower to keep it moist. You can use olive oil. But you should not put oil on your face. And mustard oil is irritating, so you shouldn't put it on your face and head. When there is too much of oil, it can coat the scalp.

You can use a low-alkali soap that is safe for your baby's skin every day. Use Sonamani shampoo on your hair twice weekly (two days is enough for newborns). After a bath, you can put lotion on the baby. But before they are 15 days old, they don't need oil or lotion. Minor children shouldn't lose their hair in the winter. Wait between 1.5 and 2 months for a baby's first hair to fall out.

Sleep safe.

Usually, a round thing like a turban is made to hold the baby's head on the bed, but this is not necessary. A soft, one-inch-thick pillow is suitable for a newborn, but make sure not to fold the neck. The square cloth for the baby can be folded to a height of one inch if you want to. After six months, the pillow can be made taller based on the child's age. At two years old, this height can be two inches. The mother will sleep with the baby. But make sure that the baby's nose doesn't get pinched by blankets, bed sheets, pillows, or even the mother's body, or that the baby doesn't fall out of bed.

Growing up

A baby should spend at least 30 minutes in the sun every day. It's best to leave it out in the sun before 9 a.m. or after 4 p.m. Mom, stay tuned. Both of them will make vitamin D in their bodies.

Hold very carefully and firmly behind the neck for three to four months. That is, the baby's head shouldn't hang down. It would help if you didn't hold the child in your lap by the hand. If you do, the shoulder joint could become loose, and the writing could hang down.Don't give walkers to teach people how to walk. In natural law, each task is conducted for the child step by step. Going against the rules can make things worse (may delay learning to walk).

You can often take the baby to the mother's office to breastfeed, and there are also places to keep the baby. If you have to, you can take the child outside.It's OK to carry the baby in front of the chest. Only he should be fully "supported," meaning his whole body should be supported.

Chapter:08

Care for babies born with low birth weights

If the baby is tiny at birth, it should stay in the hospital under the care of a paediatrician. A nasogastric tube may be used in addition to breast milk to get enough nutrition.A baby weighs less than 2.5 kg when born; it is called a Low Birth Weight (LBW) baby. If a baby is born weighing less than 1.5 kg, it is said to have a light birth weight. The baby weighs less than 750 grams and is considered highly underweight.

Many reasons a baby may be born with low birth weight. Most children born to mothers who are underage or teenagers are underweight. A baby is born early and has a light birth weight. During pregnancy, a baby may be malnourished if the mother has diabetes, heart disease, kidney disease, malnutrition, anaemia, significant infections, toxaemia, bleeding, or other problems. Babies who are twins or born with congenital disabilities can also be too small. The weight of babies born to mothers who smoke is also low.

Babies with a low birth weight get sick more often. So they need extra care. In addition, the baby's body temperature may drop after birth. So, the baby should always be kept warm after it is born. Handling the baby should be done with clean hands, and the baby should wear clean clothes. If not, the baby could get sick. If it's hard to breathe, the cold in the nose and the saliva in the mouth should be cleaned right away.

If the baby is tiny when it is born, it should stay in the hospital and be cared for by a paediatrician. A nasogastric tube may be used in addition to breast milk to get enough nutrition. The baby should be kept in an incubator if his temperature drops. Babies born before their time have trouble breathing because their lungs and other organs are not fully developed. You may need to stay in the NICU for treatment if the condition is terrible.

Chapter:09

Make exceptional food for your one-year-old.

You don't have to worry about making exceptional food for your one-year-old. Your other family members can eat them with what they eat. You have to try to eat as little salt as possible. Restaurant food is out of the question since it usually has a lot of salt.

1. Grains for food

The best always! Cereals like corn flakes soaked in milk are easy to break down. So try to eat as many cereals with whole grains as you can.

2. Cucumber

Cucumber slices are a healthy snack that can be eaten at any time of the day. The best way for your baby to eat them is to cut them in half lengthwise and shape them like French fries. On a hot day, cucumbers are an easy way to stay hydrated. can

3. Dal

Dal has a lot of protein in it, which helps build muscle. Dal-Kari can be eaten with either rice or bread, and it doesn't smell extreme. Make sure the bread is cut into pieces that are easy to eat.

4. Vegetable soup

It's easy to make for a one-year-old and has all the good things from the vegetables you put in it. In this case, carrot soup is excellent for your eyes, and potato soup has fibre in it.

5. Soya

Soy pills are another way for vegetarians who don't eat meat to get protein quickly and in good quality. It's great for kids to eat because it gets soft when it's cooked.

6. Later

It's a daily meal that everyone in the family can eat, even the kids. When you add vegetables or cheese, it becomes a well-balanced meal.

7. Chicken or meat from chicken

Make sure to buy organic chicken or chicken tested and shown to be free of hormones. Putting the chicken in the oven for a bit longer will make it more tender, which is good for your fussy baby. Also, avoid strong spicy flavours and cut cooked meat into small pieces. Then, before you give them to your baby, rip them apart and remove the bones.

8. Fish

Always remember that frying fish removes its nutritional value, which is why fish curries are not a good idea. Be very careful to take the bones out before giving your child things like chicken and other items with bones. When tearing and plucking flesh. Even tiny barbs on fish can get stuck in the throats of small children.

Make sure you have a chance to learn the following terms for a year's worth of

little gold.

1. Apple rings fried in oil(A sweet, quick snack!)

Materials

- One apple
- 1/4 cup flour
- 1/2 milligram of sugar
- A little bit of cinnamon.
- 1/2 beaten egg
- 1/4 cup buttermilk
- A little bit of salt

How to get ready

Mix the flour, sugar, salt, and cinnamon, and set aside.In another bowl, separate an egg and buttermilk and mix them.Cut the apples into slices that are 1/4 inch thick and throw away the core.Mix the two bowls of the mixture, then dip the apple rings well and deep fry them.You can also coat those fried pieces with powdered sugar for older kids.

2. Dimension

Chickpeas are high in protein, and plantains are high in carbs. Together, they make a well-balanced way to start the day.

Materials:

- Flour made from wheat
- 2 tbsp
- 1/2 of an onion cut up
- Salt to taste.
- One teaspoon of ground coriander.
- One tablespoon of coriander leaves, chopped.
- One teaspoon of garam masala,
- One teaspoon, Jowan
- 3–4 spoonfuls of oil

How to get ready

Mix the gram flour, the onion, the coriander powder, the coriander leaves, the Jowan, and the garam masala. Add oil to this mixture and knead it well to make a ball. (Do not mix water!)Make bread with the flour dough and fill it with the rice flour. Using a spoon and ghee, cook them well. Put butter or curd on them.

Chapter:10

How a 2-year-old grows and changes

When a child turns 2, there are clear signs that they are making progress. But these two-year-old milestones are just general guidelines and don't say how a child will grow. Every child grows and learns at their own pace. So, if children don't seem to have reached the expected milestones at this age, parents shouldn't worry too much or try to hurry them along.

growth of the body

Your child may be trying to use his fine motor skills to communicate better and try out new things. When a child is at the right weight for their age, most parents worry about them gaining weight. Or not. A 2-year-average old's weight can be anywhere from 23 to 28 pounds. A 2-year-body old's is likely to change in the following ways:

- He can now go up and down the stairs with ease.
- He might not have any trouble going backwards.
- By standing on his leg, he may now be able to keep his balance better, which helps him climb on anything.
- He might also be able to draw circles and other shapes.
-
- He can now hold his favourite crayon with his thumb and some of his other fingers.
- He will now be able to put his building blocks together to make a tower or bridge.
- With some help, your little one can now put on some of his clothes again.

The 2-year-old child's social and emotional growth

- Your child might now be ready to share with a friend or sibling, but this isn't always the case. Even if he has a friend to play with, he may still prefer to play by himself. For example, the following changes in social and emotional life A child of 2 years old might see:
- A child this age might sometimes act like an older child and want to be treated like a younger child. This kind of emotional conflict is typical at this age, and it could get worse if he changes his routine. For example, she wants or expects you to show her more love and attention.
- At this age, your child starts to notice that boys and girls are different. For example, a little boy might want to walk or dress like his father, while a little girl might want to do everything her mother does, even if it's her father. The mother might be busy trying to put on her favourite lipstick.
- Also, kids can often choose not to act like their "ideal" person of the same sex. The same goes for this. Children's minds are naturally curious and like to try new things.
- Your baby might not worry too much about being away from you.
- Your baby may have a few times when they don't listen or get angry at this age.

Language and thought development

- At this age, your child may be able to point to balloons, dogs, balls, etc., in pictures in a book, but he may not yet be able to understand abstract ideas. Some of the things that happen during cognitive and language development are:
- Your child might like to pick out things independently and put them in groups.
- He might start to repeat a sentence by using a few phrases.
- As he learns more about himself differently, he may be able to say what he likes and doesn't like.
- He will be able to understand and do what is asked of him.At this age, your child may ask "why" a lot. He might say it when he wants to know the truth about something. And sometimes, he says it out of the blue because he doesn't know how else to show how interested he is. going to
- At this age, your child may start to understand words like "hurry," "late," "good," and "bad."

Act in a set way

- At this age, your child may become very hard to please. He might want things a certain way and get angry if they don't turn out that way. So you might hear some whining or "pan-pan" every time. He might also not like being turned down or told no.
- Children sometimes fuss again because they are hungry or tired. Taking care of these two issues could make him less fussy. Sometimes, kids may feel stressed or want your attention again. You can, most of the time, stop these meltdowns by cuddling them or making them feel better. You can also keep your child busy by giving them exciting toys or getting them involved in something fun.

Chapter:11

Social and Emotional Growth :

3 to 4 years old —

- At this point, they discover that they must communicate with many individuals besides their mother, father, brother, and sister. The first stage of socializing begins. Their inner world is quite strong. They cannot discriminate between false and genuine work. They can not comprehend whether witches do magic or whether youngsters may transform into birds and fly. At this age, children do not lie. However, kids frequently conflate fiction and reality.

- By the age of three, children learn that their minds are distinct from those of their parents and that they cannot read their minds.

- Comprehends the meaning of large and tiny, as well as long and short. But they cannot be separated. For example, a quick, thick glass can contain more liquid than a tall, thin glass.

- As night follows day, one discovers their age.

At this age, he is learning how to draw. Most have large, spherical heads and long legs that begin below the eyes. Learn how to draw squares and crosses. Can construct a bridge with three bricks.

Years five and six:

- The first person to comprehend the significance of friendship. She wants to cultivate and play in the field with friends.

- Attempts to assist mother with minor duties. The interest in toys declines while the interest in living things increases. Spends considerable time with a cat or dog as a pet.

- Time for the first hand of chalk. Learned to interpret letter meanings. A child learns to write words within three months of mastering the alphabet.

- Learned how to create paper boats, planes, and other objects and desires to do it himself.

What to avoid:

Children are for love; this must be remembered. However, it should not be forgotten that teaching children the correct ideals would not satisfy their unwarranted desires.

Many adults do not listen attentively to children. Do not comprehend how vital it is to answer their minor inquiries.

- For instance, by frightening the ghosts - if you don't do this, the snail will come and bite you, or if you pass under the tree, the spirit will lay eggs - these thoughts must never reach the head. Teach him to be resilient in the face of life's numerous obstacles. If you instil fearful thoughts in a child at a young age, he will be unable to let go of many things as he matures.

- Children can often utter a great deal of gibberish and irrelevant statements. Explain it courteously without becoming annoyed or amused.

The majority of mothers place their hands on their children. Indeed, discipline is essential, but it should not be extreme. Explain patiently and without excessive repetition. Express to your youngster your love for him. You will gain from it. The youngster will consider your input when making meaningful choices. You will be an indispensable component of his life.

- Never force a situation. Children are an integral part of you. Think of him as a part of you. Avoid projecting your aspirations onto him.

Instead of negative behaviours today, practice eating a balanced diet. Children don't even want to eat. Do not force yourself; eat slowly and patiently.

- Parental conflict and separation ruin the child's mentality. So raise children together and pay close attention to one another. Your love will inspire them to love as well.

In the following situations, a physician's guidance is crucial:

- Care should be taken to ensure that youngsters are growing appropriately. A skilled paediatrician should consult a height and weight chart organized by age for infant girls and boys. Determine if his growth is proportional to other children at the appropriate age.

- Take it seriously if a task now requires more time than in the past. Observe whether he is consistently sliding into this issue.

- Frequently, a child's body swells and accumulates water due to protein deficiency caused by severe malnutrition. Consult a physician immediately if you experience anaemia, vomiting frequently, or vertigo.

Some infants are born with congenital physical deformities. Please do not interfere with them, and inform your doctor. Many diseases are curable if diagnosed and treated at a young age. Don't wait to get older.

Every parent adores their child. Similarly, this adorable infant should be cared for. Therefore, maintain your health and shower your child with affection.